STAYING AWAY FROM CANCER: ALL YOU NEED TO KNOW ABOUT CANCER

BY

DR. JENNIFER GODWIN

Copyright@Dr.Jennifer Godwin

All right reserved

TABLE OF CONTENTS

INTRODUCTION

Chapter one

Cancer cells and normal cells

Chapter two

How cancer develop

Chapter three

Types of cancer

Chapter four

Signs of cancer

Chapter five

Preventive measures of cancer

INTRODUCTION

Malignant growth is a sickness wherein a portion of the body's cells develop wildly and spread to different pieces of the body.

Disease can begin anyplace in the human body, which is composed of trillions of cells. Regularly, human cells develop and duplicate (through an interaction called cell division) to shape new cells as the body needs them. At the point when cells become old or become harmed, they kick the bucket, and new cells have their spot.

Once in a while this deliberate cycle separates, and unusual or harmed cells develop and duplicate when they shouldn't. These cells might frame growths, which are chunks of tissue.

Growths can be carcinogenic or not malignant (harmless).

CHAPTER ONE
CANCER CELLS AND NORMAL CELLS

Harmful growths spread into, or attack, close to tissues and can head out to far off places in the body to frame new growths (a cycle called metastasis). Carcinogenic cancers may likewise be called threatening growths. Numerous malignant growths structure strong cancers, however tumors of the blood, like leukemias, for the most part don't.

Harmless cancers don't spread into, or attack, close by tissues. At the point when eliminated, harmless cancers ordinarily don't bounce back, while destructive growths now and again do. Harmless growths can now and then be very enormous, nonetheless. Some can cause serious side effects or be hazardous, like harmless growths in the mind.

Difference between cancer cells and normal cells

Cancer cells contrast from normal l cells in numerous ways. For example, cancer cells:

fill without even a trace of signs advising them to develop. Normal l cells possibly develop when they get such signals.

disregard flags that typically advise cells to quit separating or to pass on (a cycle known as customized cell demise, or apoptosis).

attack into neighboring regions and spread to different region of the body. Typical cells quit developing when they experience different cells, and most ordinary cells don't move around the body.

advise veins to develop toward cancers. These veins supply growths with oxygen and supplements and eliminate side-effects from cancers.

stow away from the safe framework. The safe framework regularly kills harmed or strange cells.

stunt the safe framework into assisting disease cells with remaining alive and develop. For example, some malignant growth cells persuade invulnerable cells to safeguard the cancer as opposed to going after it.

collect numerous progressions in their chromosomes, for example, duplications and erasures of chromosome parts. Some malignant growth cells have twofold the typical number of chromosomes.

depend on various types of supplements than typical cells. Furthermore, some malignant growth cells make energy from supplements another way than most ordinary cells. This lets disease cells develop all the more rapidly.

CHAPTER TWO
HOW CANCER DEVELOP

Disease is a hereditary infection — that is, it is brought about by changes to qualities that control the manner in which our cells capability, particularly the way that they develop and separate.

Hereditary changes that cause disease can happen on the grounds that:

of mistakes that happen as cells partition.

of harm to DNA brought about by unsafe substances in the climate, for example, the synthetic compounds in tobacco smoke and bright beams from the sun. (Our Malignant growth Causes and Counteraction area has more data.)

they were acquired from our folks.

The body regularly wipes out cells with harmed DNA before they turn malignant. Yet, the body's capacity to do so goes down as we age. This is essential for the justification for why there is a higher endanger of disease sometime down the road.

Every individual's malignant growth has a remarkable blend of hereditary changes. As the disease keeps on developing, extra changes will happen. Indeed, even inside similar growth, various cells might have different hereditary changes.

CHAPTER THREE
TYPES OF CANCER

Carcinoma

Carcinomas are the most widely recognized kind of disease. They are framed by epithelial cells, which are the cells that cover within and outside surfaces of the body. There are many kinds of epithelial cells, which frequently have a segment like shape when seen under a magnifying instrument.

Carcinomas that start in various epithelial cell types have explicit names:

Adenocarcinoma is a malignant growth that structures in epithelial cells that produce liquids or bodily fluid. Tissues with this sort of epithelial cell are at times called glandular tissues. Most diseases of the bosom, colon, and prostate are adenocarcinomas.

Basal cell carcinoma is a disease that starts in the lower or basal (base) layer of the epidermis, which is an individual's external layer of skin.

Squamous cell carcinoma is a malignant growth that structures in squamous cells, which are epithelial cells that lie just underneath the external surface of the skin. Squamous cells likewise line numerous different organs, including the stomach, digestion tracts, lungs, bladder, and kidneys. Squamous cells look level, similar to fish scales, when seen under a magnifying lens. Squamous cell carcinomas are here and there called epidermoid carcinomas.

Momentary cell carcinoma is a disease that structures in a kind of epithelial tissue called temporary epithelium, or urothelium. This tissue, which is comprised of many layers of epithelial cells that can get greater and more modest, is tracked down in the linings of the bladder, ureters, and part of the kidneys (renal pelvis), and a couple of different organs. A few malignant growths of the bladder, ureters, and kidneys are temporary cell carcinomas.

Sarcomas are tumors that structure in bone and delicate tissues, including muscle, fat, veins, lymph vessels, and sinewy tissue (like ligaments and tendons).

Osteosarcoma is the most well-known bone disease of bone. The most widely recognized kinds of delicate tissue sarcoma are leiomyosarcoma, Kaposi sarcoma, dangerous stringy histiocytoma, liposarcoma, and dermatofibrosarcoma protuberans.

Leukemia

Malignant growths that start in the blood-framing tissue of the bone marrow are called leukemias. These diseases don't shape strong growths. All things being equal, enormous quantities of strange white platelets (leukemia cells and leukemic impact cells) develop in the blood and bone marrow, swarming out ordinary platelets. The low degree of typical platelets can make it harder for the body to get oxygen to its tissues, control dying, or battle diseases.

There are four normal sorts of leukemia, which are gathered in light of how rapidly the sickness deteriorates (intense or persistent) and on the kind of platelet the malignant growth begins in (lymphoblastic or myeloid). Intense types of leukemia develop rapidly and persistent structures develop all the more leisurely.

Our page on leukemia has more data.

Lymphoma

Lymphoma is malignant growth that starts in lymphocytes (Immune system microorganisms or B cells). These are illness battling white platelets that are important for the insusceptible framework. In lymphoma, strange lymphocytes develop in lymph hubs and lymph vessels, as well as in different organs of the body.

There are two primary kinds of lymphoma:

Hodgkin lymphoma - Individuals with this infection have strange lymphocytes that are called Reed-Sternberg cells. These cells normally structure from B cells.

Non-Hodgkin lymphoma - This is an enormous gathering of tumors that beginning in lymphocytes. The diseases can develop rapidly or gradually and can shape from B cells or Immune system microorganisms.

Our page on lymphoma has more data.

Different Myeloma

Different myeloma is a disease that starts in plasma cells, one more sort of safe cell. The strange plasma cells, called myeloma cells, develop in the bone marrow and structure cancers in

bones generally through the body. Various myeloma is likewise called plasma cell myeloma and Kahler illness.

Our page on numerous myeloma and other plasma cell neoplasms has more data.

Melanoma

Melanoma is malignant growth that starts in cells that become melanocytes, which are specific cells that make melanin (the shade that gives skin its tone). Most melanomas structure on the skin, yet melanomas can likewise frame in other pigmented tissues, like the eye.

Our pages on skin malignant growth and intraocular melanoma have more data.

Cerebrum and Spinal Line Cancers
There are various kinds of mind and spinal string growths. These growths are named in view of the kind of cell in which they framed and where the cancer originally shaped in the focal sensory system. For instance, an astrocytic growth starts in star-molded synapses called astrocytes, which assist with keeping nerve cells sound. Cerebrum

growths can be harmless (not disease) or threatening (disease).

CHAPTER FOUR
SIGNS OF CANCER

Signs and side effects brought about by disease will differ contingent upon which piece of the body is impacted.

A few general signs and symptoms related with, yet not well defined for, disease, include:

Weariness

Bump or area of thickening that can be felt under the skin

Weight changes, including accidental misfortune or gain

Skin changes, for example, yellowing, obscuring or redness of the skin, injuries that will not recuperate, or changes to existing moles

Changes in entrail or bladder propensities

Constant hack or inconvenience relaxing

Trouble gulping

Roughness

Constant heartburn or inconvenience in the wake of eating

Constant, unexplained muscle or joint torment

Industrious, unexplained fevers or night sweats

Unexplained draining or swelling.

Conceivable Gamble FOR Malignant growth

Your age

Disease can require a long time to create. That is the reason the vast majority determined to have disease are 65 or more seasoned. While it's more normal in more established grown-ups, malignant growth isn't solely a grown-up sickness — disease can be analyzed at whatever stage in life.

CHAPTER FIVE
PREVENTIVE MEASURES OF CANCER

Certain approach of life choices area unit glorious to make your gamble of malignant growth. Smoking, drinking over one food daily for girls and up to 2 beverages per day for men, spare openness to the sun or incessant rankling burns from the sun, being stout, and having dangerous sex will boost unwellness.

You can address these propensities to bring down your gamble of malignant growth — but many propensities area unit additional easy to alter than others.

Know Your case history

You inheritable over your mother's eyes or your father's grin. they will even have shared their possibilities for having diseases like cancer. Some genes that folks pass right down to their youngsters have flaws. they do not repair broken DNA the approach they must, that lets cells become cancer. study your family's medical record and raise your doctor if a genetic check may be a smart plan for you.

Avoid cytotoxic Chemicals

Chemicals referred to as carcinogens harm DNA in your cells and lift your likelihood of getting cancer if you bit, eat, or breathe them in. Asbestos, radon, and benzol area unit many that some individuals acquire contact with at work or home. Chemicals in weedkillers, plastics, and a few home merchandise may additionally be risky. you cannot avoid each chemical, however recognize which of them area unit in merchandise you utilize and switch to safer choices if you'll.

Loose many Pounds

Extra weight around your middle may add up to a bigger likelihood of getting cancer, particularly of the breast, colon, uterus, pancreas, esophagus, and bladder. Researchers say one reason is also that fat cells unleash substances that encourage cancer cells to grow.

Avoid Smokes

Every puff of tobacco is packed with 250 harmful chemicals. Nearly seventy of them cause cancer. And it's over simply carcinoma. Cigarettes area unit joined to twelve other forms, together with abdomen, bladder, kidney, mouth, and throat. the earlier you stop, the better. raise your doctor for recommendation on quit-smoking strategies.

Eat additional Broccoli

Fruits associated veggies pack an anti-cancer punch as a result of they are high in nutrients and fiber, and low in fat. attempt broccoli, capital of Belgium sprouts, cabbage, kale, watercress, or different dilleniid dicot family vegetables. They defend against DNA harm which will flip cells cancerous. Or eat colourful berries. Studies show they need cancer-fighting chemicals that keep at bay harm to cells.

Get Off the Couch

Do you pay an excessive amount of time unerect around? Cancer hindrance is an extra reason to urge moving. Exercise fights avoirdupois and lowers levels of hormones like steroid hormone and internal secretion, that are joined to cancer. Aim for half-hour of cardiopulmonary exercise -- the type that gets your heart pumping -- on most days of the week.

Go straightforward on Alcohol

Tip back too several martinis day after day, and your odds of cancer go up. Alcohol is joined to cancers of the mouth, breast, liver, esophagus, and others. The additional you drink, the upper your risk. If you drink, have sex carefully. ladies ought to persist with one drink daily, men up to 2.

Cut Back on Hot Dogs

Think twice before you throw some on the grill. Studies show that processed meats, like hot dogs, bacon, and sausage, have chemicals referred to as nitrites and nitrates that will be joined to cancer. And analysis suggests an excessive amount of pork like cut and burgers might be a semipermanent risk for large intestine cancer. select safer alternatives for your curtilage picnic, like malformation or fish.

Put on ointment

Baking within the sun may offer you a healthy-looking glow, however beneath the surface, ultraviolet light rays cause skin harm that would result in cancer. as a result of you'll burn in precisely quarter-hour, rub on ointment before you go outside. choose a broad-spectrum product with associate SPF of thirty or higher. Reapply whenever you sweat or swim. And once you are call at the sun, wear a wide-brimmed hat and garment eyeglasses.

Practice Safer Sex

Sexually transmitted diseases (STDs) are not your solely worry throughout unprotected sex. a number of these infections conjointly increase your odds of getting cancer. concerning seventieth of cervical cancers begin with human papillomavirus (HPV) varieties sixteen and eighteen. Some forms of infectious disease will cause liver disease. to remain safe, use a latex rubber on every occasion you've got sex.

Get unsusceptible

When it involves vaccines, assume on the far side your annual contagion shot. Some will defend against cancer, too. sure HPV vaccines stop cancers of the cervix, vulva, vagina, and anus. The time to urge unsusceptible is between ages nine and twenty six. The hepatitis B immunogen wards off the virus that causes liver disease. It's a part of the childhood vaccination schedule.

Stay Up thus far With Screenings

Screening tests catch cancer early -- typically even before it starts. A endoscopy typically finds polyps within the colon and body part before they become cancer. The Papanicolaou test locates pre-cancerous and cancerous cells in a very woman's cervix. Mammograms and low-dose CT (LDCT) seek for early breast and respiratory organ cancers. raise your doctor once to begin obtaining these tests, and the way typically you would like them.

www.ingramcontent.com/pod-product-compliance
Lightning Source LLC
Chambersburg PA
CBHW050324220526
45465CB00005B/2124